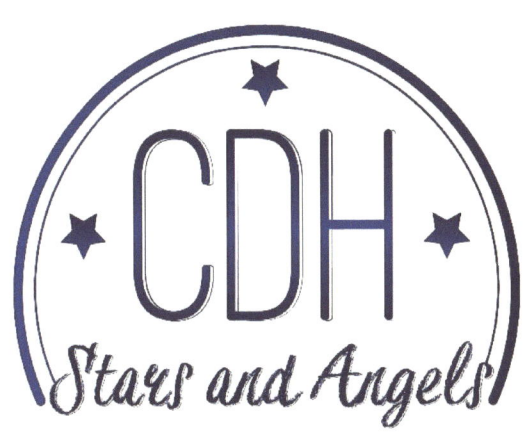

Congenital Diaphragmatic Hernia Awareness
Spring 2018

Copyright © 2018 Brenda Mertes

All rights reserved.

ISBN-10:1717239404
ISBN-13:9781717239402

CDH Awareness Bridge Weeks:

One organization holds their awareness day on March 31st. Another holds theirs on April 19th. CDH Stars & Angels bridged the two dates for our first annual CDH Awareness Bridge Weeks. During these weeks, we held several giveaways and activities. We are grateful to those who participated as well as the businesses that donated and made it possible to have a wonderful event.

Among the events we held, we made live videos and shared our stories. We also shared pictures, and taught strangers about this birth defect. Then there were the giveaways, which were truly awesome!

WonderWorks in Orlando, Florida donated two tickets to their laser tag arena, which were given to one of our affected families. Premier Cancun Destinations also generously donated a resort stay to one of our very deserving families who has done so much for the CDH community. We look forward to hosting this again next year as the organization grows.

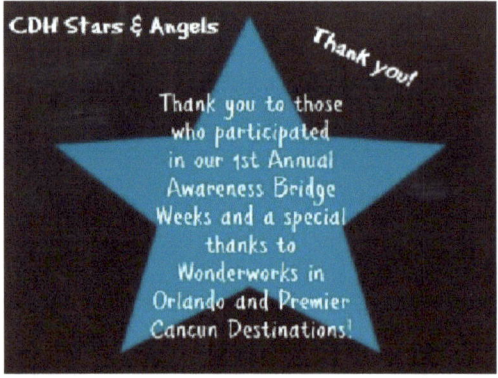

Garrett's story:

Soon after my 20 week ultrasound I got a phone call that I was being referred to a high risk OB because my son had a diaphragmatic hernia. They couldn't get me in for awhile so I did a Google Search on it because I had never heard of it before. My son has a life-threatening birth defect. I was devastated, wondering what I did wrong, how this happened, and wondering what was going to happen next. My first appointment was a very long one. I had another ultrasound, met with a genetic specialist, had an amniocentesis, and then finally talked to the OB. They told me that he had a 10% chance of survival and if any abnormalities came back from the amnio then there was no chance of survival and I could deliver anywhere because he would not make it.

I decided to get a second opinion because I didn't want to accept the fact that I might lose my son. The new OB/ surgeon/ NICU team gave us an 80% chance of survival.

On April 26, 2016 Garrett was born. They whisked him away into the next room so they could start life-saving measures. On their way out of the operating room I got a quick glimpse of him before they took him to the NICU. I had no idea what was going on. Two long hours later they brought him into my room so I could see him before they transported him to the Children's hospital. My husband went with him so that if the worst case scenario happened he wouldn't be alone.

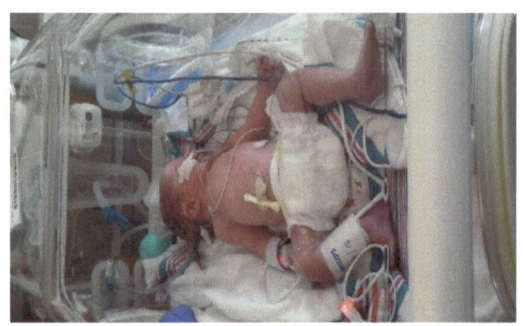

I was discharged two days later right before his repair surgery so I was able to touch him and love on him before he was taken into the operating room. After his surgery he was in the NICU for a week and then was transferred down to the regular hospital floor. There they started the process of weaning off of oxygen and starting feeds. After a total of six weeks and two days in the hospital, he was discharged! He came home on oxygen support and a feeding tube. The first few weeks were very challenging trying to take care of such a medically complex baby but we got through it! He is no longer on oxygen but still has a feeding tube due to aspirating. He has weekly physical, speech, and feeding therapy. Through this journey he is one of the happiest and strongest kid that I know. You would never know by looking at him that he began his life fighting for it. He has definitely changed my life for the better!

-DeAnn Hamilton

FAMILY FINE LINES

"My mother thinks I just don't trust her."

I've heard this line a hundred times. Having a baby with Congenital Diaphragmatic Hernia is not easily relatable (fortunately) and therefore, it is common for family members to not understand why we take certain precautions with our little ones. In the aftermath of repair surgery, relationships suffer because family and friends start to feel that they can't visit their loved one in the hospital for personal reasons. Most of the time this isn't true.

There are limits on how many visitors that a baby in the neonatal intensive care unit can have. This is to prevent an overwhelming amount of people in one room at a time and potential illnesses. Even the parents of babies in the NICU are forced to stay away from their little one if they are coughing or feverish. Whether it is a grandparent, sibling, extended family, or friend that gets to visit is also up to the parent but very limited.

Once the baby is discharged, it is very important for the family to have little interaction with anyone for a short while. Bringing a severely ill infant around a lot of people immediately after hospitalization poses a huge risk for their fragile immune systems. Extended family, church members, co-workers, family friends, and neighbors should respect the precautions taken by parents of CDH babies for the sake of their fragile lives.

Moreover, anything as simple as a respiratory infection could end the lives of a CDH survivor. Lung growth is hindered when abdominal organs float into the chest cavity through the hole in the diaphragm. This is definitive of Congenital Diaphragmatic Hernia. Thus, these children and older survivors have fragile bodies and take risks when they are in public schools, daycares, playgrounds, in the workplace, and in stores. Germs are everywhere!

It is part of our role to inform the public of the risks that they and their families take with the lives of those who are medically fragile, when they go to church and other public places when they are sick themselves. It is not an exaggeration to say that it could literally end the lives of Congenital Diaphragmatic Hernia survivors.

Things You Need To Hear:

1. **You are NOT alone!** While the diagnosis of Congenital Diaphragmatic Hernia occurs in 1 in every 2,500 live births, having a special needs child or a medically fragile child is not a rarity.

2. **Take care of you!** The guilt that parents of CDH babies put on themselves when they leave their child's bedside in the NICU for even moments...really weighs on how capable they are of coping with the reality of the situation and being able to further help take care of their little one.

3. **Make Therapy Fun!** One thing that therapists tend to do is to make physical therapy and speech therapy FUN. Children then may see therapy as play and not just another doctors appointment. On the other hand, play is therapeutic as well. Engaging in regular crafts and activities with your little one teaches them important developmental skills.

4. **It is not your fault!** Too many parents of CDH babies or special needs children in general, blame themselves. If you're asking yourself what you did to cause your child suffering – stop. The cause of CDH is unknown and there is nothing you could have done to prevent it.

5. **You will have to make life-altering decisions for your child!** There is no way around this. Parents of "normal" babies make life-changing decisions for their children when they decide what their child is going to eat, where they are allowed to play, how they dress, who they are around...your job will be a little tougher than that. Some days you'll have to decide whether your child does enroll in speech therapy, you'll feel guilt if you don't register them immediately. There will be times when you will be asked if you want your child to have a scary test performed "just in case" there is something wrong with them that wasn't caught in previous testing. Again, the guilt will be immense if you don't agree

to it. Take care of yourself and know that it is better safe than sorry. Also realize that if you are doing the very best that you personally can for your child and have chosen doctors that you ultimately trust – then there is nothing else that you can do.

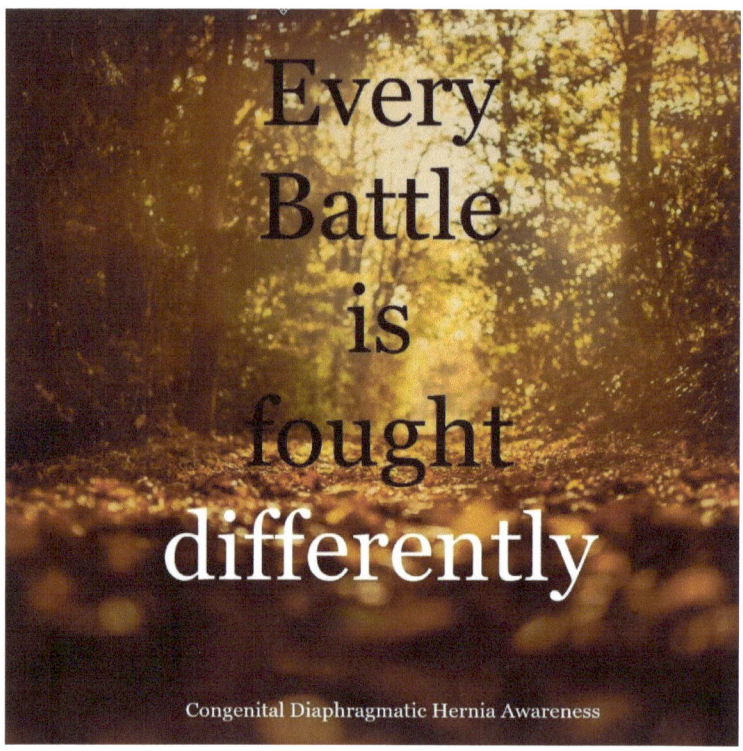

Long-Term Effects of CDH

CDH Survivors live with long-term medical problems. Respiratory issues are generally common among CDH children and adults, but there are other issues such as possible reherniation (when the patch covering the hole in the diaphragm reopens), Pectus Excavatum (the breastbone sinking in and hindering heart and lung function), bowel obstruction, bleeding in the brain, behavioral issues, and vision and hearing loss. Occasionally babies born with Congenital Diaphragmatic Hernia also have illnesses such as Trisomy, Autism, Congenital Heart Defects, and more.

It is also common for CDH survivors to not meet their developmental milestones for their age. Parents of survivors therefore spend a lot of time taking their little one to physical therapies, speech therapies, CDH clinics, and regular pediatric appointments to try to get their child to the appropriate developmental stages. Some parents feel that this has robbed them of time that could have been spent registering their child for sports, fun hobbies, and any social activity. Being around other parents who have babies without medical issues and who can participate in regular activities, is emotionally difficult.

When the parents of these survivors take precautions and set boundaries with family members, it is a necessity and not spite.

Emery Hadden's Miracle Birth

At 20 weeks pregnant I went to my normal ultrasound to get a sonogram. They told me they were transferring me over to a high risk doctor because they were 99.9% sure my unborn daughter had CDH. They started telling me about it and told me that she wouldn't live. According to them, she only had a 5% chance and for us to basically be prepared. That I would push her out, hold her, and they would take her away to paralyze her and sedate and give her morphine. So on August 14th, miracle baby girl – Emery Kate Hadden – made it into the world. As soon as i pushed her out she was blue and wasn't breathing or crying. They took her right away and incubated her, paralyzed her and gave her morphine to start her feeling comfortable. Within four hours she was already on ECMO, which she needed it in order to survive. Well, ECMO saved her life. She was on that for fourteen days.

After coming off that she still had the vent down her throat and was always just swollen, laying there & doped up. On August 31st (two days after getting off ECMO) she had the repair. It was successful. She had just enough muscle on the rim of the diaphragm to attach the patch to be able to survive. She fought for her life for 40 days. She suddenly made a turn around and started doing better, got off all the medicines, they took her off the vent and put her on cPAP. After a week they tried the regular nasal cannula.

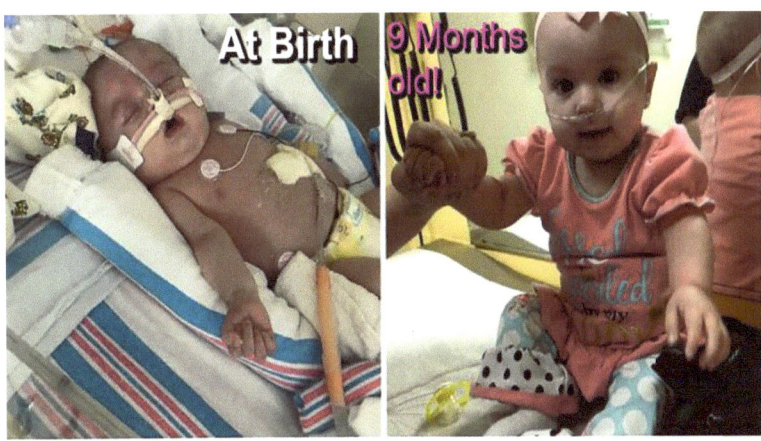

In the midst of all this, we did get to hold her for the first time on day seventeen. What a joy!! She had two brothers. One was two years old and the other one was five. The five year old got to meet her, but the two year old didn't until she came home. I stayed with her lots of nights, being restless and just wanting to know my baby was okay. On day 52 a miracle happened and she got to come home. She never learned how to suck a bottle or eat. She came home with an NJ tube & oxygen. Still to this day she has oxygen and on March 9th we got her a g-tube through the stomach. Way less stress for here at home & she is starting to talk a lot more now. She's nine months old now and doesn't roll over, crawl, talk or do things like a normal nine month old would do. She's delayed and takes speech therapy, occupational therapy, physical therapy and early intervention every week to try to catch up! We are glad she's here and living today. ECMO machine definitely saved her life, as well as the doctor that did her repair surgery. My baby is a miracle and still fighting today! She kicked CDH BUTT. She has to take tons of medicines each day, and they're saying she will have another surgery in August 2018.

-Destiny Hadden

HOPE = HEALTH

Life really changes with just a sentence.

"Your baby has Congenital Diaphragmatic Hernia."

"If you abort now, you will probably have a healthy pregnancy later."

"We can't find your baby's heart."

These are all real quotes from ultrasound technologists and doctors. The doctors then ask if you have any questions or concerns, but the only thing you really want to ask is, "why?"
...and there is no answer. There is no known cause.

However, there is hope.

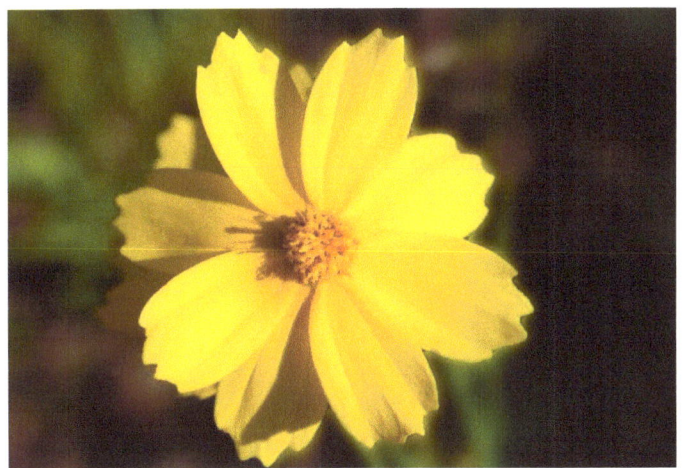

Recent studies from universities such as Harvard have shown that optimism is key to getting through just about anything. Those who have a brighter outlook are normally people who lead healthier lives and are generally happier. Health, hope, happiness, and optimism are all interchangeable.

How is this relevant to CDH?

When expecting parents receive the news that their child is very ill and has Congenital Diaphragmatic Hernia, it feels as if their baby has just been given a death sentence. When these parents are prepared for what could happen but still have hope and recognize the possibility of their little one surviving, they lead healthier lives and are emotionally more capable of coping with the reality of the situation.

When parents unfortunately face the devastating loss of their child, it is necessary to get through the beginning stages of the grieving process. This isn't a process that will ever really end for these parents. Holding onto the hope that their child's story will inspire other parents and let other grieving parents know that they are not alone, allows for grieving parents to cope better.

When older survivors are optimistic about the procedures that they have already been through and may face in the future, hanging onto the recognition that they have already survived more than a lot of people could, they too can better face the reality of their futures and know that there is a future for them. These studies also show that those who are more optimistic tend to live longer, which has some obvious implications for CDH survivors.

In addition, one study found that there is a link between emotions and viral infections, blood pressure, and heart attacks. In the study, doctors found that pessimists are three times more likely to have a heart attack. Given that survivors of Congenital Diaphragmatic Hernia already have heart and respiratory problems, it is very important for them to also have hope.

We don't encourage false hope. We don't encourage anyone to disregard the possibilities with CDH. This is a life-threatening birth defect and we have heard the stories ranging from the least severe cases to the most severe, as well as stories of parents who have had multiple CDH survivors and angels. We do encourage hope because we want families that are affected to be able to cope with this diagnosis as well as they possibly can. CDH Stars & Angels and its leaders are not experts on this birth defect, but rather parents who have went through it on different levels ourselves and want the world to know all about it.

Board Game Donation Day!

This is a project we are working on in honor of a CDH survivor that gained her wings this year. She loved board games and was very competitive. It was almost the only thing she had to do during lengthy hospital stays. We realize that there must be many more patients at children's hospitals that also have lengthy stays with little to do and we are collecting brand new, unwrapped board games for them.

On June 9th, one administrator and I will spend all day at a local courthouse to collect all board game donations.

On the day listed below (May 14th, 2018) present your ticket to your server at Buffalo Wild Wings. Ten percent of your total bill will be donated to CDH Stars & Angels Inc.

13882 Bell Rd.
Surprise, AZ

11 AM – 11 PM

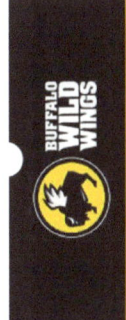

EAT WINGS. RAISE FUNDS.

On the day listed below, present this ticket to your server and Buffalo Wild Wings® will donate 10%* of your total bill (not including tax, gratuity or promotional discounts) to our organization.

Buffalo Wild Wings strives to support our community and the organizations and sports teams within it. Together we can make a positive impact and help keep our community working and playing together.

(Show this ticket to your server on the date & time listed below.)

CDH STARS & ANGELS
May 14, 2018 • 11:00 AM - 11:00 PM
13882 W Bell Rd. • Surprise, AZ • 623-546-7672

ADMIT ONE

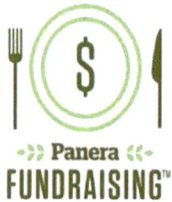

Panera FUNDRAISING

HELP SUPPORT

CDH STARS & ANGELS

WHERE 3550 South Highway 528 NW, Albuquerque, NM 87114

WHEN Mon, Jun 25th **FROM** 4:00pm - 8:00pm

Bring this flyer or show an electronic version to the cashier when you place your order and we'll donate a portion of the proceeds from your purchase.*

Ordering Online for Rapid Pick-Up or Delivery?*

Enter "FUND" as your Promo Code to have a portion of your proceeds donated to your organization.

Learn more at **PaneraBread.com/fundraiser**

*Gift card purchases and catering orders are excluded and will not count toward the event. Rapid Pick-Up and Delivery only where available.

© 2018 Panera Bread. All Rights Reserved.

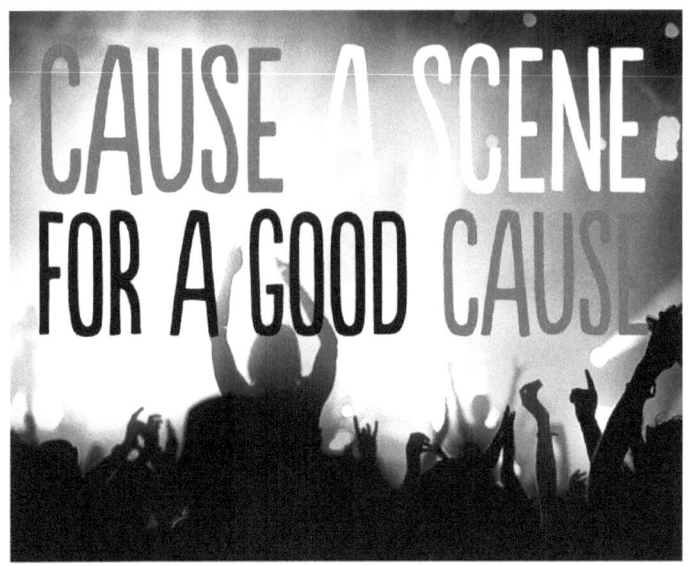

Enjoy yourself and support our cause at a special fundraising event for:

Organization name: CDH Stars & Angels Inc.
July 12th, 2018
Blaze Pizza
Gainesville
3617 Archer Rd.
Gainesville, FL 32608

Bring in this flyer or show it on your phone before paying. Blaze Pizza will donate 20% of proceeds from your meal back to our organization.

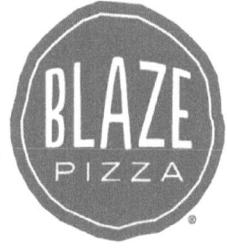

FAST·FIRE'D®

Donation amount excludes proceeds from tax and gift card purchases. Valid for dine-in and take-out only. Not valid for online orders. Alcoholic beverages excluded. Event proceeds void if flyers are distributed in or near the restaurant.

Blaze Pizza (Gainesville)

3617 SW Archer Rd, Gainesville, Florida 32608

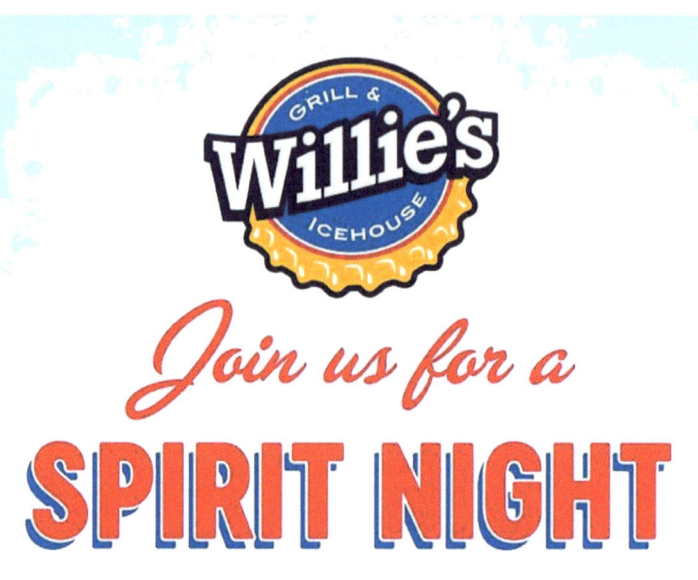

Join us for a
SPIRIT NIGHT

TO BENEFIT

CDH STARS AND ANGELS

WHEN	WHERE
TUESDAY, JUNE 19, 2018 4PM - CLOSE	ALL LOCATIONS

MENTION YOU ARE DINING IN SUPPORT OF
CDH STARS AND ANGELS
& WILLIE'S WILL DONATE **15%** OF YOUR CHECK

ACKNOWLEDGMENTS

1. DeAnn Hamilton (Garrett's Story)
2. Destiny Hadden (Emery Hadden's Beginning)
3. Paula Crites (Sunflower Photography)

www.ingramcontent.com/pod-product-compliance
Lightning Source LLC
Chambersburg PA
CBHW040312220526
45473CB00002B/638